I0421364

Spring Renewal
Heart Healing for the Mind, Body and Soul

Amy Zielinski

This book is dedicated to all beings everywhere, across time and space. May we each experience, honor, and celebrate all of our transitions.

Cover art: "High Country Lavender"
Artist: Karen Wallace
From the private collection of Kareen Lopez

www.divineunion.us

Table of Contents

Heart Healing and Renewing our Relationship with Ourselves

As the striking clock heralded the new millennium on New Year's Eve 2000, I was writing my wish for the coming year onto a piece of paper that I then folded and placed into a special box.

"I want my heart to grow larger and more open," I wrote. I was referring, of course, to my metaphoric heart ~ what I perceived as the storehouse of my emotions, the gateway through which I interacted with other humans, the seat of my compassion and love. It was *that* heart that I wanted to experience as more spacious and open.

Within eight months, however, I would learn that my *physical* heart was, indeed, growing larger and more open; this organ had become greatly enlarged due to a rare and deadly condition and I would soon undergo open heart surgery in an attempt to save my life.

It appeared that I had received my New Year's wish . . . in ways that I am still uncovering today

My physical heart changed entirely during that serious heart and lung illness; however it did not change nearly as much as my *real* heart did. During this period, I learned to open and experience life in ways I had never done before. My *relationship* with my heart was entirely new, which led to all of my relationships becoming renewed. Because of this, I can never view this physical condition as creating "heart damage" in me ~ rather, it grew and healed my heart, perhaps even birthed a new heart.

It was this experience that opened my awareness to the heart's immense capacity for healing ~ both for healing itself and for being the source of healing for all of the relationships in our lives. Conscious use of the heart's capacity for healing allows us to continually renew and recreate our relationship to all aspects of our being ~ our bodies, minds, and souls.

Spring Renewal

Like the Earth, all living beings experience seasons of birth, growth, decay, and death ~ continually. And this means that our relationship with each aspect of our being is constantly changing. We do not relate to our minds or our emotions the same ways we did as toddlers. Renewing our relationship to our bodies, minds, and souls occurs throughout our lifetimes ~ sometimes without our awareness and sometimes with great consciousness.

Even as the Earth creates room for fresh growth each Spring, our beings generate space for new opportunities (jobs, relationships, homes) by releasing those that no longer serve us. We are continually experiencing the death of Winter so that we can participate in the births of Spring.

But Spring Renewal isn't just for spring; it is what happens when we transition from the end of one phase to the birth of another ~ the end of a relationship calls for Spring Renewal, as does the beginning of a new career. When we move into a new home, we can use the benefits of Spring Renewal, just as we can when our physical bodies experience change brought about by aging or illness.

Heart healing practices are the foundation of a conscious approach to renewing and healing ~ no matter what areas of our lives are in need of renewal and healing.

Heart Healing Practices

Our hearts are not merely blood-pumping muscles located at the center of our physical bodies. They are also the centers of many elements of our lives. We connect to our deepest integrity by "crossing our hearts", we have integrated something mentally when we "know it by heart", and when we feel something strongly we do so "in our   hearts."

Indeed, the center of anything ~ a tree, a country, a family, a situation ~ is referred to as its heart ("the heart of the matter", for instance). This centrality is not just about the location of the heart; it also describes the importance of the heart. The heart of anything is its most essential component.

When we work to heal anything from its central, most essential core, that healing energy radiates outward to all other parts of the organism or situation. Just as physical hearts send healthy blood to every part of our physical body, our hearts also have the capacity to send healthy energy to every part of our being ~ to our bodies, minds, and souls. Even as our bodies have immune systems that function to heal whatever physical ailments we may have, from a skinned knee to advanced stages of serious disease, the immune system of our entire being is our heart. In fact, our hearts are able to send healing energy well beyond our own beings ~ to other humans; to the Earth on which we live; indeed, to all beings everywhere.

Plenty of systems discuss healing one's relationship with the body or the mind or with another human. What, exactly, is it that is doing that healing? The heart. And what is the vibration the heart emanates? Love.

This love is not merely a warm feeling of affection or fondness; it is an actual energy, a vibration, that each of us has the capacity to generate, to send forth, and to receive. Each of those actions ~ generating, sending, and receiving love ~ is integral to heart healing. And each one involves practice.

Heart healing is not just conceptual. It is a body of practices that are rooted in our physical and spiritual heart centers. These practices heal and connect us to all aspects of our being and to all of our relations.

"How will my heart know where to send the blood?" I wondered after waking up from a life-saving surgery that provided me with a new pathway between my heart and lungs. "What if it keeps trying to go the old way?" I asked my amazingly patient surgeon.

Taking out his model of a human heart, he described to me how blood always takes the path of least resistance. My heart would quickly realize that this new pathway was a much better channel through which to send blood into my lungs to be oxygenated. "Pretty smart," I thought.

Just like water finding its way around stones and trees and other obstacles, blood finds its way . . .

. . . and so does love.

But this requires that we actually practice sending that love where we want it to travel. We can keep our regular old pathways going, even though they may be corroded or narrowing or tightening due to neglect or grievances or stubbornness. Or we can work to create all kinds of new pathways.

This process of building new love tunnels is an ongoing one, one that requires consistent practice. Sometimes I feel like I am back in the operating room, carving new pathways and opening up existing ones, as I learn how to expand my heart even bigger and how to keep increasing the ways love flows from it and to it.

It is not sufficient for us to think about love or to talk about the experience of heart healing. This unparalleled healing ~ healing that radiates outward from our very core to all aspects of our being and beyond, to other humans and all beings everywhere ~ only happens when we actually engage in heart healing practices. This book will introduce you to and guide you through such practices so that you can use them to renew your relationship with your body, mind, and soul.

This volume is a guidebook of sorts ~ a grouping of articles that detail how I approach heart healing and renewing my relationship with all different aspects of my being.

The entire book can be followed like a step-by-step field guide on a journey toward healing and renewal of your relationship with your body, mind, and soul. This is particularly helpful during major life transitions, such as losing a job or becoming a parent.

You may also choose to use this volume as a reference book ~ to explore heart healing as it relates to the renewal of one or more particular aspects of your being.

I have included suggestions for practices at the end of each chapter. These are offered as inspirations rather than assignments. Choose those that compel you and integrate and adapt them into your life in whatever ways are most healing and renewing for you.

This offering comes with a blessing and a prayer: may we each return again and again to our center ~ our heart ~ to experience the healing power of our own love and radiate that outward to all aspects of our being and to all of our relations.

Heart Healing Practices

Altar: Create an altar dedicated to your heart and to its immense capacity to heal and renew all your relations. Spend time with your altar, connecting with your your heart.

Nature as Teacher: Spend some time outdoors, connecting your heart essence with the heart essence of something in nature ~ the Earth, a tree, a four-legged being or a winged one, for example. Once you begin to experience this connection, imagine radiating it outward in all directions.

Sitting Practice: Sit in a comfortable position, breathing deeply and fully into your heart. Place your awareness on the center of your chest, imagining that you can breathe into your heart. With each breath, begin to explore your own heart essence ~ what does *your* heart feel like? Once you connect with this essence, radiate it outward throughout all parts of your physical form.

Spring Inspiration for Heart Healing and Renewal

Clean Monday.

Is that some new Happy Homemaker Holiday implemented to celebrate how tidy our homes are or to herald the period when we reseal our grout tile and polish metal door and window hardware, as prescribed by Martha Stewart herself? (Yes, there is, indeed, available online a checklist of such duties, should you choose to use it.)

Nope, that isn't what Clean Monday is about; at least, not exactly . . .

In Greece, Clean Monday is celebrated each year during the seventh week before Easter. I first encountered this holiday as a teenager living in Athens and was mildly curious about why we were given a break from school for cleaning ~ on some Monday or any other day, for that matter. What I began to learn those many years ago was the importance ~ and antiquity ~ of cleansing rituals performed during the late winter and spring months, the cleansing of living environments as well as the deeper cleansing of our bodies and spirits.

The Greeks are not alone in performing purification rites during this time of transition between winter and spring. Many western Christians celebrate Lent by purifying their bodies through dietary fasts and abstentions, and Jews may prepare for Passover by scouring their homes for any crumbs of *chametz* and then burning this leavened bread while eating only unleavened bread or *matza*. The Iranian New Year occurs around the time of Spring Equinox, and for millennia people in this region have commemorated this time of year by thoroughly cleaning their homes. Before Christianity arrived in Greece, spring was the time for purifying the temple of Athena in Athens; the idol of the goddess was removed, her home was scrubbed and ridden of all impurities, and the deity's statue was then taken in a procession to the sea, where it could be washed as well. We also have a great deal of evidence for similar spring cleansing ceremonies held throughout northern Europe thousands of years ago.

So, could Clean Monday, Passover purification rituals, and ancient spring rites have anything to do with Martha Stewart or with the February or March issue of any home and lifestyle magazine, which usually remind us that this is the time to "De-Clutter Your Life"? Absolutely!

Spring Cleaning. This phrase may call to mind your grandmother or her mother taking rugs outside to beat them in the fresh air or your parents pulling everything out of the garage in an annual attempt to rearrange the same stuff in the same space. Maybe you recall helping to clean the windows; perhaps you have your own cleansing rituals that you perform in and around your home each year.

For thousands of years, people have devoted a large amount of energy to cleaning each spring – cleaning their homes, their fields, and their bodies. This is often necessitated by lifestyles. In agrarian communities, the fields have to be prepared before planting can be done. Some homes shelter farm animals during the colder months and can finally be returned fully to their human inhabitants during this time of year. In households that have not been opened during the winter months, debris from heating elements and tremendous amounts of very stagnant air can finally be removed. And spring's warmer weather provides a welcome chance to catch up on tasks that may be precluded by winter's cooler temperatures, such as the washing of windows and walls.

Although many of us are blessed with tools that make our cleaning jobs much easier and more pleasant than were those of our ancestors, we are no different from those who have come before us in our urge to scrub our homes each spring. The desire we have to clean our environment and the satisfaction that we feel once we have done so are the same desire and satisfaction they felt. These rituals we perform with our mops and soap and brooms are age-old; they are age-old, because they are entirely in alignment with the earth and with the changing of the seasons. It seems natural for us to want to clean during the spring. We feel the newness in nature all around us and want to bring that into our homes and our lives as well. As the tiny crocuses pop up out of the earth to herald that another winter is passing, we feel the desire to push past the debris of fall and winter and blossom ourselves. We begin to feel the extra energy of more daylight hours in our bodies, and we see the energy of emerging life around us; we can pull all this new energy in and apply it to tasks like cleaning our homes.

And for perhaps just as long as people have been cleaning the places where they live each spring, they have chosen this time of year to cleanse themselves. This seems to me to be purely natural. The earth cleanses herself; windstorms in early spring freshen the top soil so that buds may more easily pop through the earth's surface. Just as the earth needs to be rid of the old in order to make room for the new, we do too.

Like the earth, many of us spend the winter months turning inward. Just as the earth is not "dead" during winter, we are not gone or even merely resting; instead, we are in a sort of psychological and spiritual pregnant phase ~ a time when things may be growing underneath the surface, even as we appear on the outside to be very still and calm. Although our bodies may be somewhat dormant, they are doing very hard work, very important work. No, it is not the work of summer, which is active and obvious and full of fiery passion. It is the work of winter, of nurturing things that are growing under the surface. These things will sprout during spring and grow during the summer . . . but they will grow much better if we have prepared our fields.

So, how do we do this type of preparing? What exactly are we renewing? And what tools do we use for jobs that obviously cannot be completed with mops and rubber gloves?

Fortunately, our ancestors as well as countless contemporary spiritual practices provide us with supplies and equipment for this Spring Renewal.

During this period of preparation for and celebration of new life, we can focus on the renewal of our beings, specifically in different realms: mental, spiritual, emotional, and physical.

And if that all sounds a bit daunting, we can again look to Greece for inspiration.

You see, in addition to cleaning out their homes on Clean Monday, Greeks also spend time doing something that seems to have nothing at all to do with Spring Cleaning; they go in large masses to the countryside to picnic and fly kites. Why? Because this cleaning they ~ and we ~ are beginning is a joyful practice, one that brings us closer in communion with the divine, one that allows space in our lives for us to blossom as the gorgeous spring flowers we are.

So, no special paraphernalia is needed for this cleaning; just some curiosity, an open heart . . . and perhaps a picnic basket full of yummy food and a kite!

Spring-Inspired Practices for Heart Healing

Altar: Create an altar dedication to Spring. Include any objects that signify renewal and rebirth. Spend time at your altar, connecting with the healing energy of Spring.

Nature as Teacher: Dedicate some time to finding and exploring evidence of the continual renewal that occurs in the natural world. Find examples of all phases of life ~ birth, grow, decay, and death ~ all around you.

Prayer/Blessing: Create or find a prayer or blessings that honors renewal and rebirth. Use it daily to anchor your connection with these healing energies, connecting with the energy of your heart as you repeat the words.

Celebration: Pack a picnic and a kite and spend a day outdoors, celebrating the healing and renewing that is to come.

Facing our Demons: Lions and Tigers and Bears, Oh My!

So, here we are with a relatively large renewal project in front of us; how should we approach it? Let's imagine that it is a many-roomed house. Should we bounce from room to room, organizing a bit here and there and then moving onto another room as the mood strikes us? Maybe . . . That may be a fun approach, but I do not have a very high success rate with that method.

Nope, I have learned from years of experimenting that my projects need to be broken down into manageable bits; I must focus on one piece of the project, one room of the house or even one drawer in the dresser, at a time. So that is the way I work with Spring Renewal ~ the healing of all aspects of my being. I break this healing project into different sections, focusing on one specific realm of my being at a time. And I invite the healing properties of the four elements to help me renew that aspect of myself.

From Ancient Greek to contemporary Wiccan customs, from Far Eastern Asia to North America, countless peoples have turned to the four elements of nature for inspiration and understanding of their own beings. Air, fire, water, and earth are the building blocks from which are constructed all life forms on our planet ~ including us. And in many different belief systems, these elements are each associated with a different realm of our being. Air can be seen to represent our mental body, Fire our spiritual body, Water our emotional body, and Earth our physical body. Each element is also associated with a different cardinal direction, a specific season, a time of the day, and a plethora of symbols. These various traditions and associations can ~ and will ~ provide us with much information, insight, and guidance as we work to heal and renew these aspects of our lives.

We do not need, though, to consult any esoteric texts or visit any gurus in order to access the four elements in our Spring Renewal. We can find inspiration for our healing in what may be a much more assessable, if somewhat unorthodox, source. The film *The Wizard of Oz* has been a brilliant teacher for me regarding these aspects of my "self". Each of the characters on the journey to find the Wizard believes that he or she is lacking in a specific area of his or her being. The Scarecrow feels he needs a brain (mental); the Lion, courage (spiritual); the Tin Man, a heart (emotional); and Dorothy, a home (physical).

As the four journeyers set out, each feels somehow deficient. And each learns, of course, that everything he or she perceived as being absent was there all along. When the Wizard presents the awards, we are made aware of the Scarecrow's intellect, the Lion's bravery, and the Tin Man's huge capacity for love ~ all things that each always had, things that had to be remembered and reclaimed. The journey itself is what allows these strengths to be seen; it is as though the powers each character has are uncovered bit by bit with each step along the yellow brick road, with each demon faced.

Just like these well-loved characters, we also take that journey and face demons as we discover, purify, and reclaim the power of our mental, spiritual, emotional, and physical beings. This process of learning about our own power is precisely what we are doing when we renew these different aspects of our being.

And for many of us, discovering our own power and perhaps learning to use it in healthy ways seems every bit as frightening as the journey throughout Oz. Just think about it: perhaps you sometimes hear a cackling, witch-like voice admonishing you in your head for some perceived wrong-doing; maybe you have worries of releasing flying monkeys if you were to ever get in touch with emotions you've stored away for decades; and the lions and tigers and bears you fear threatening your safety could be changes in your health, income, or partnership status.

Just like our counterparts on the silver screen, many of us may place our hopes in some Wizard who will provide us with all we need, who will make up for whatever deficiency we feel we have. If you've ever entertained thoughts like, "I will love my body once I lose _____ pounds," or "When I make $_____, then I'll feel safe," or "That new book or class or spiritual practice will provide me with clarity and peace," you've been in search of your own Wizard.

And, like Dorothy and her friends, you've probably come to know that such a Wizard was really just some guy hiding behind the curtain, wielding controls for fancy sound and lighting effects, a "humbug".

So, a vital element in reclaiming our power and living authentically involves pulling back that curtain and discovering what is hiding in our mental, spiritual, emotional, and physical beings. And aspects of that can seem really frightening at first.

Each of us has renewal work we consider to be really easy and others that feel incredibly daunting; and these are not the same for any two people. Sometimes what determines whether we consider a job pleasant and simple or difficult and challenging are purely its physical requirements; some of us do not enjoy working in the yard, while others dislike spending time in small spaces like closets.

In my experience, though, the jobs that we repeatedly shy away from are those that may not be as physically arduous as they are mentally, emotionally, or energetically demanding. These tasks have enormous "pulls" for us, associations that make the cleaning job not just about the physical aspect of cleaning.

Many of us avoid cleaning specific areas of our homes (or offices or cars or finances) because we are afraid of what we will find there. For years, I avoided cleaning my craft closet. I kept all the other closets in my home beautifully organized, and I welcomed the tasks required for this maintenance; however, I felt huge resistance every time I approached this specific space. Why? Was it because it was more physically challenging to clean than my other closets? No, it was because I knew that it would be difficult to find what was there. I did not want to see what I had been storing there, because I knew that I would use that information against myself. I would see projects I had not finished and berate myself for not finishing them. They would become further evidence in the ever-mounting case of Amy Not Finishing Things She Begins.

The thought of cleansing and revitalizing our mental or emotional beings may be every bit as scary as was cleaning my craft closet, because we worry about what we will find in these realms of our being.

Sometimes we choose to hang onto things in our living environments that no longer serve us and that may actually be detrimental to us. For instance, some people choose to keep old clothes that no longer fit or suit them in case these will someday fit, thinking, "Maybe I'll lose ten pounds and be able to wear those pants again." So each time they choose their daily outfit, they must rifle through pieces that are not currently being used, pieces that are not serving them. In the case of ill-fitting clothing, this causes not only a misuse of time but it can be emotionally draining as well, if it can provide an impetus to scold ones' self for the ways a body has changed. Similarly, as we do our Spring Renewal, we may come across things that we've kept that no longer serve us, things we actually use against ourselves. Just like those skinny jeans from high school, it is time to clear all that out!

Occasionally, we may hoard memories or grudges or emotional baggage . . . just in case we need them in the future. And we may kid ourselves that we do not really focus on them as we push them out of the way in our daily lives. But just like those old jeans, they register with us each day as we scurry past them, trying to avert our eyes and ignore them.

Have you ever kept an item that really did not serve you, simply because you had invested a large amount of money on it? We frequently hang onto relationships or behavioral patterns that are unhealthy for us, merely to honor the weighty investments we have made in them; and we wait around for some kind of return on that investment.

None of this hanging on serves us ~ in our closets

or in our lives. But in order to rid our beings of those things that no longer are beneficial to us, we first have to acknowledge them. And that can feel a lot like facing the Wicked Witch of the West. Once we do this, though, we may just find that all it takes is a bit of water to melt them away.

When Glinda the Good Witch explains to Dorothy how to return home, she says, "You've always had the power to go back to Kansas." The Scarecrow questions her, "Then why didn't you tell her before?" And Glinda answers, "Because she wouldn't have believed me. She had to learn it for herself."

We all have always had the power to be fully whole; indeed, we already are. But no one can tell us about it, because we cannot believe. We have to learn it for ourselves.

And here's how we start . . . we just follow the yellow brick road.

<u>Heart Healing Practices for Facing our Demons</u>

Altar: Create an altar to the Four Elements (Air, Fire, Water, and Earth) and to the aspects of yourself that each represents (Mental, Energetic, Emotional, and Physical). Spend some time with your altar, honoring the gifts of each element your relationship to it.

Nature as Teacher: Dedicate some time to exploring the classroom of nature. Use each of the elements as your teacher: be open to the gifts and wisdom they share with you and how these can be utilized in your healing and renewal.

Sitting Practice: Sit comfortably and breathe deeply into your heart. One by one, witness the current state of each aspect of your being: mental, energetic, emotional, and physical. Without judgment or a need to fix or change anything, simply notice what that part of you is experiencing in this moment. When discomfort arises, send the healing energy of your heart to the part of your being experiencing the discomfort.

Media Inspiration: Watch *The Wizard of Oz*. Celebrate as the characters each realize that they already have that which they were seeking. Celebrate your own wholeness and perfection in this moment!

Meet Your Backup Singers: Spring Renewal of the Mental Body

One recent weekend morning, I was curled up in bed, enjoying the cozy feel of a Sunday without plans, as I watched my partner bending over my laptop. The previous evening, I had clicked on the wrong button, causing the screen to freeze, and he was investigating the possible damage. I could feel his anxiety level rise as the virus scan came back with some warnings in red, "Infestation! Epidemic!!" His body began to hunch over and his heart began to close as he read these warnings. "This doesn't mean that our computer *has* a problem, merely that it *may* have a problem," I suggested in what I hoped was my most reassuring voice. He didn't seem comforted; in fact, what I thought was a helpful contribution seemed to annoy him . . . perhaps because it momentarily distracted him from his state of worry – one to which he felt quite accustomed.

So I did what I often do in such situations ~ I became playful. I jumped out of bed, started be-bopping around the room, and in my best doo-wop back-up singer voice, sang, "Doom and gloom . . . and doom and gloom . . . and doom and gloom . . . ." This had its intended effect, as he was eventually able to laugh, sit up a bit more straightly, take a few deep breaths, and realize that the world was, in fact, not about to end. This possible infestation, this epidemic, would not, it seems, be the end of us. (And by the way, my computer was just fine!)

You see, his Backup Singers are the Doom and Gloom Guys and Gals. For decades, they have been punctuating many of his experiences with their admonitions that things are about to go terribly, horribly awry.

The chorus usually performing in my mind is a different one, of course. Rather than flashy, boisterous lounge lizards, I have a group of very quiet and subtle, sweet-voiced little singers who whisper to me in an enchanting melody, "Hide; stay small; be safe. Hide; stay small; be safe," as they tiptoe around. They always appear when they sense that I am living into my truth, opening up to the bigness of who I am, and their soul purpose is to convince me not to do that, to hide my light from others in order to be secure.

Who are your Backup Singers? What is the chorus they continually repeat in your head? Many of us have several tracks available to us, and we turn to the appropriate one for each situation. Bank account a bit low? No problem, let's use the "Danger, You Will Soon be Living on the Streets" blues number. For the times when a relationship ends, we can always turn to the, "You Will be Lonely Forever" melody, and every time we make a mistake we can strike the chords of the "You are Never Right" overture.

I was not always aware of this singing going on in my head. That awareness came through time spent watching my mind with curiosity, which is exactly what I invite you to do. Each of us has songs or soliloquies or arguments running through our minds, and most of the time we cannot even really hear them; they form a continual, background chatter that flows endlessly on and on in a loop throughout each of our days. The trouble with that is that they can have a tremendous amount of power over us. They can have really appealing voices, which are sometimes booming and loud and other times more soft and subtle; or perhaps they sound a bit scary. If we look closely, we will find their origins in the voices and words of our childhoods. You may hear your parents or teachers or friends in these choruses. Sometimes it is helpful to locate those voices to learn where they originated; however, it certainly is not essential.

What *is* essential is bringing those words and songs out into the light, acknowledging their presence.

Why? If we just ignore them, won't they just go away?

Not in my experience. I have found that the less we know about them, the more powerful they are. So we must get to know them.

Let's play with this a little bit:

1. Call to mind a worrisome situation, either real or imagined.
2. Make it as real as possible and go fully into the feeling state that you associate with this situation.
3. Now, observe your mind for five minutes.

What did you notice? Did you hear any singing, or yelling, or nagging? That was your mind. And guess what? It was almost definitely lying to you.

Yes, my friends, I did just call your mind a liar; but no, I most certainly did *not* call *you* a liar. It is vitally important that each of us not only understands this distinction between our minds and ourselves but also accepts and honors this differentiation. We are much, much bigger than our minds. They are very useful tools; however, they are only tools.

And, in fact, our Backup Singers ~ our minds in general ~ are quite frequently liars.

I knew that my partner's Doom and Gloom Guys and Gals are liars, because none of their predictions of upcoming horribly catastrophic events had ever materialized. The late night when he could not reach me on my cell phone and they began to sway him with their siren song of disaster, they were wrong (I had merely forgotten to charge my phone battery).

And my Backup Singers are no more trustworthy than his; the only dangers I have really faced have not ever been brought about by me living into my truth. Rather, it has always been following their siren-song advice to "hide and stay small" that has invariably led me astray.

No noise could be heard from our Backup Singers during times of real peril. When my partner was in dangerous situations during his deployment to Iraq, his mind was absolutely focused on what had to be done; there was no extraneous mental chatter at all. When I felt myself becoming very ill, I had absolute mental clarity around what actions needed to be taken and how to approach my healing.

Why? Where do these "clear thoughts" come from? They come from a place that is much more expansive than our minds, and each of us has had the experience of having them ~ or hearing them, or feeling them, or knowing them ~ throughout our lifetimes. By focusing on healing and renewing our relationships with our minds, we create space for these "clear thoughts", these experiences of true knowing, to guide our lives. Just as a garden needs to be weeded in order for healthy plants to take roots and grow, our mental bodies must be cleared of the debris lurking there ~ the chatter of our Backup Singers that threatens to overtake the fertile soil of our minds.

Meditation is the surest way I (and countless people throughout the ages) have found to really get to know what the mind is doing. It does not require hours and hours spent in some stiff posture, trying to "clear" your mind or someone whacking you with a stick each time you seem to be drifting into thought (although both of these experiences are available to you, if you desire to create them). The practice of meditation simply asks of us that we get quiet for a bit of time and notice what happens. Simple, right? Yes, very simple; and hardly easy. What usually happens is that we sit down and begin to watch our thoughts . . . and they then come flooding in: What am I going to make for dinner? It feels warm in here; I wonder if we'll have an early Spring? I think maybe I upset my brother when we talked yesterday . . . and on and on. That's okay!! When we continue to watch, we learn priceless information. We are then able to see whether we spend more time focusing on the past or on the future, we watch ourselves create worries and fantasies, and yes – we meet our Backup Singers.

There are many other practices that can help us with Spring Renewal of the Mental Body. Going into silence is an invaluable method for observing our minds as we begin this cleansing. But a practice of silence does not require you to retreat to a cave somewhere for ten years.

How about two hours without reading, writing, speaking or listening to any words at all? Or perhaps you can decide that tonight when you go to that cocktail party you will refrain from telling any stories about yourself or anyone else?

These practices are a lot like cleaning out the garage, in that they can get pretty messy before we get to the bright, sparkly clean part. They allow us (indeed, they force us) to focus our awareness on our thoughts. Without the constant noise of television news and songs on YouTube and chitchat in the grocery store aisles, we can now focus entirely on our Backup Singers. And when we decide to spend some time refraining from talking about ourselves, our stories, and our pasts, we may finally notice a nice little piece of mental clutter to investigate. Now that we have shined the light on it, we can get to know it and decide wether it is something we would like to keep or release.

The element we associate with our mental beings is Air, and it is so useful to turn to both the element and its symbols for inspiration as we heal and renew our relationship with our mental bodies. Meditation teachers often suggest that new practitioners envision their minds as the open sky with their thoughts passing through as clouds.

We need to remember, though, that clouds are not

always puffy, cotton candy balls of fluff that float lazily along. Sometimes they are low and dark and threaten to burst forth with torrential rains at any moment.

Similarly, our thoughts come in all different forms. And, just like clouds, they eventually pass.

The time of year we associate with this element is the Spring, with all its new birth and freshness everywhere, and the time of day related to this element is the morning. As we focus on noticing any clutter that may be stored in our mental beings this week, let's be encouraged by the newness of the day and of the season. Our minds have the same capacity to ceaselessly begin anew; we need merely create some space for our new thoughts ~ healing, loving thoughts ~ to be born.

Once we shine the spotlight on our Backup Singers, we may find that they are actually kind of harmless and funny. And now that we have brought their choruses to center stage, we are at choice about what to do with them. We can continue to let them drone on and on in the background all day long . . .

. . . or we may decide to teach them a new tune.

Heart Healing Practices for the Mental Body

Altar: Create an altar to healing and renewing the relationship with your mental body. Incorporate any objects that you associate with this healing and renewal, including symbols of the element of Air. Spend time with your altar, connecting with your intent for healing and renewal.

Nature as Teacher: Dedicate some time to communing with the element of Air. Be open to any gifts of wisdom you may be given and integrate these into your healing and renewing of the relationship with your mental body.

Sitting Practice: Breathe deeply into your heart. Begin to witness your mind; what types of thoughts arise? When you notice a thought, without judgment or a need to change or fix anything, simply direct (using your breath and your imagination) energy from your heart to your brain, picturing your heart essence bathing your mental body.

Meet your Backup Singers: Devote some time to getting to know your Backup Singers. When are they most active? What is their tune? Once you feel intimate with them and their siren song, you may choose to reclaim some of the power this tune has taken from you over the years by creating a song-and-dance routine inspired by it. Each time you feel your Backup Singers beginning to warm up, externalize the tune ~ have fun with it rather than succumbing to its negative message.

All Fired Up: Spring Renewal of the Energetic Body

This little light o' mine
I'm gonna let it shine
This little light o' mine
I'm gonna let it shine
This little light o' mine
I'm gonna let it shine
Let it shine, let it shine,
Let it shine.

~ Harry Dixon Loes

The association of our energetic or spiritual beings with the element of fire is age-old and ubiquitous and can perhaps be seen most readily in our use of language. Someone is "all fired up" when he or she is passionate about something. The "spark of inspiration" touches us and compels us to move forward on a project or to create a way out of a difficult situation. And if we cannot find this spark, perhaps someone will help to "light a fire under" us.

Just like fire, the intensity available in our spiritual beings has all different flavors. Sometimes, we may feel a steady, warming fire similar to that in a hearth; on other occasions, our spirits feel more like roaring bonfires. There are occasions when our energy seems akin to an out-of-control, raging forest fire; and other periods when we may swear we can only feel a slight flicker of candle flame glowing in our energetic being.

Each of these fiery essences may be useful for different purposes; my goal through Energetic Spring Renewal is to have at my disposal a flame that I can use in whatever way I want. Once I have healed and revitalized my relationship with my energetic being, I am then able to build this fire into whatever level of intensity I desire to use at any point.

We all know that fires must be cultivated and tended in order for them to be useful. If our fuel sources are unclean, our fire may produce harmful smoke. If we forget to add fuel when needed, our fires can quickly become extinguished. And a fire ~ even a small candle ~ left unattended may become uncontrollable and even dangerous.

How can we heal and renew our relationship with our energetic beings so that we are able to consistently care for these fires that fuel our lives? There are three steps that are essential in this process, and they are steps that we need to repeat consistently throughout our lives (in other words, this renewal is a lot like all other forms of renewal ~ it is an ongoing process!):

1. Claiming our Fire

2. Purifying our Fire

3. Celebrating our Fire

Get to Know Your Own Magic (Claiming)

My daughter woke up one morning soon after her first horseback riding adventure, wanting to ride a horse again RIGHT NOW! She ran around the house, frantically searching for something that could stand in for a trusty steed. As her gaze fell on a broom, her entire face lit up. She had found her horse! She asked her father to fashion reigns for her horse, which he attempted to do from an old piece of rope. She played delightedly for awhile; however, when the rope slipped and her "reigns" disappeared, she fell apart. With that slippage, the illusion that she had been swimming, dancing, and playing in had fallen apart. She screamed for help and let him know that he HAD to fix it correctly if she was going to be able to play horse again.

At that moment, my sweet daughter made a mistake, and this mistake had nothing to do with ropes or brooms, but everything to do with her spirit. She had confused the location of the energy behind her imaginative play. She thought that the rope being perfect held all the magic. She thought that it was her dad who turned the cleaning tool into a galloping stallion. She was absolutely wrong; the magic was in her from the beginning. *She* was the one who could look at a broom and see a horse. Her fire, her magic was the power at work; not her father's, not the broom's.

Don't we all do this, in one way or another? Do we give away the keys to our magic by not even really understanding our own power in the first place? So often we think that other people, certain situations, and specific sacred objects bring energy to our lives, rather than realizing that the fire of our energy, of our spirit, burns in us alone and requires no one and nothing other than itself to blaze brightly.

The first step of healing and renewing our relationship with our energetic bodies requires us to get to know them. So I invite you to spend some time just exploring and experiencing your energy. What is your particular flavor of fire? What's your magic?

Does your fire ask that you express it in large, very physical ways, like dancing and running around? Or is your fire a steady and consistent slow-burning flame? Is it easy for you to feel the spark of your spirit . . . or are there blocks that seem to complicate your access to it?

You may find that your energy comes in large waves of creative outbursts punctuated by periods of rest and calm. Many of us have experienced huge expansions of our energetic beings that are then followed by contractions. Nothing you experience is wrong or bad; it merely is.

Our first step in Spring Renewal of the Energetic Body is to get curious about our own energy and to begin honoring it by expressing it in ways that feel good to us. Shout! Dance! Make art! Make mud pies!

Play in the fire of your own spirit!

Burn Only Clean Fuel (Purifying)

My laptop computer often has a very sweet little message for me: "You are now running on reserve battery power." And I chuckle each time I see those words, because I am very aware that at times, like my computer, I also am running on "reserve" power. There are occasions when my spirit, my energy, seems much depleted and I must recharge it, just like I do my computer.

What kind of fuel do you burn best? Perhaps quiet time spent in nature feeds your spirit. Maybe reading inspirational books or collaborating with a friend or a partner is what builds your fire.

Just as some foods can be better fuel for our bodies than can others, there are some sources of fuel that are better for our energetic bodies than others. Although certain activities ~ watching edgy, dramatic television shows or gossiping with a friend ~ may give us a momentary burst of energy, they can leave us feeling like we do during the eventual drop following a caffeine and sugar-induced double-mocha-latte high.

Once you have gotten to know what the fire of your energy feels like, the next step in cleaning it involves really investigating the burning materials you feed it. For one day, take inventory of all the activities you do and rate your energy level both before and after each one. I have done this activity for weeks at a time, and it never fails to provide me with an incredible amount of useful information ~ sometimes very surprising information.

And your results may surprise you too! Perhaps you have always known that talking on the telephone drains you; but maybe you will see that talking with specific people about certain subjects actually increases your energy. Or you may learn that it is not the entire chore of laundry that causes you to lose steam, but merely the putting away of clothes that takes a good chunk of your energy.

All of this data is incredibly useful when we decide to purify our energetic bodies, because we can clearly see what helps to build our fires and what dampens them. It would be lovely if we were then able to never do any activity that lessened our energy again; this is not the case for most of us. However, we can now decide to schedule our days so that we are managing our energy better. By doing this, we can keep our battery charged more often; and when we do need to go into our "reserve power," we have a list of activities ~ our reserve batteries ~ that are the cleanest and most efficient ones for us to use.

Stay Out of Someone Else's Fire Pit – and Keep Others Out of Yours (Celebrate)

I spent six months driving with a friend to a once-a-week class that met about an hour from where we both lived. This seemed like a wonderful arrangement, because we could catch up with one another and save gas money at the same time. It eventually became apparent to me that I needed to choose between two types of energy to "save": the energy that fueled my car and the energy that fueled me. After really tracking our conversations, I realized that my companion was siphoning off my energy, much like you would gasoline from a car's gas tank. She continually listed for me things that I "needed" and told me what I "should" do; this process seemed to really energize her, but it always left me feeling very tired. Gas prices can get really high, and sharing driving responsibilities helped with my family's budget. However, my own energy prices can be even higher, and the budget of my spirit is ultimately much more important than that of my bank account.

There are countless ways that individuals try to pull on each other's energy, rather than relying upon their own. We may notice someone's fire burning brightly and toss a harmful remark their way in order to dampen their spark and hopefully attract a bit of it to our fire.

Sometimes we see that someone has a tremendous amount of light and we try to suck some off for ourselves by treating them as our unpaid therapists or personal ministers, believing that if we just have a bit of whatever fuel they have got going we will be able to allow our fires to burn brightly. And sometimes we notice that those around us have flames that are different from ours ~ brighter, dimmer, whatever ~ and we hide our own fires for fear that they will be disruptive to others.

The final step in Spring Renewal of the Energetic Body is to celebrate our own unique fires by keeping them clean, pure, and entirely our own. Notice when spending time with specific people makes you feel flat. And then STOP spending time with them! Be aware of the times when you need a person or situation to help get you feeling fired up, and then go back again and again to your own flame, your own magic, and . . .

Claim your fire!
Purify your fire!
Celebrate your fire!

LET YOUR LIGHT SHINE!

Heart Healing Practices for the Energetic Body

Altar: Create an altar to healing and renewing the relationship with your energetic body. Incorporate any objects that you associate with this healing and renewal, including symbols of the element of Fire. Spend time with your altar, connecting with your intent for healing and renewal.

Nature as Teacher: Dedicate some time to communing with the element of Fire. Be open to any gifts of wisdom you may be given and integrate these into your healing and renewing of the relationship with your energetic body.

Sitting Practice: Breathe deeply into your heart. Begin to witness your energy in this moment: is it edgy? Sluggish? Scattered? Dissipated? Notice that your energy body may feel very small or very large and that it may change in size and feeling frequently. There is no need to change or shift your energy; simply become aware of it. Next direct energy from your heart outward to your entire energetic body, offering gratitude for the ways you are served by it.

Energy Tracking: Spend a day tracking your energy. Notice what activities and interactions give you energy and which ones drain you of energy. What kind of fuel are you using? Are you staying in your own fire pit? Simply observe your own fire in all its fluctuations throughout the day. With the information you glean, you may device a plan for more efficient energy-usage in the future.

Contents Under Pressure: SpringRenewal of the Emotional Body

The beginning of school can be a really challenging time in our household. My children's anxiety levels rise as they meet their new teachers and friends and adjust to different schedules and the academic and social demands of a new year. They are each able to negotiate this new level of stress during the school day; however, once they are comfortable in our home, they feel safe articulating the energy, emotion, and anxiety they are feeling. These expressions are often quite loud, and they are occasionally directed at their beloved family members. Since I am always around, that usually means I am on the receiving end of these expressive outbursts.

I have worked very hard over the past several years to refrain from taking these emotional expressions personally. I realize, for instance, that the genesis of my daughter's anger when she screams, "Where is a *good* pencil? We don't have *anything* I need in this house," is probably not the presence or lack of a writing implement. Likewise, I am quite certain that when my son cries, "You never listen to me; you love her more," as his sister interrupts a conversation, he is not actually questioning my devotion to him. On most days, I am fully aware that they are communicating feelings that have been bottled up during the course of their day, and I have the presence of mind and the openness of heart to help them find the sources of these emotions, investigate them, and ~ most importantly ~ to express them.

On some days, though, my mind is not clear, my heart is not open, and I cannot seem to find one bit of patience with which to handle their outbursts. One such morning, my daughter was expressing a huge amount of anxiety on our way out the door by obsessing about the way her shoes felt on her feet and complaining that her brother was talking too much and yelling that I was not giving her the answer she wanted to whatever question she had raised. I felt an enormous amount of anger building inside of me, and ~ rather than express it verbally ~ I slammed my car door in rage.   This slamming unhinged something in the door mechanism (and in me!), causing the car then to not open from the inside. I could not get out of the car through the driver's door; I had literally imprisoned myself by my own repressed anger!

It took me a few moments to realize the hilarity of the situation; once I did, I began to laugh hysterically at my predicament, as I wondered just how many times through the years (hundreds? thousands?) my repressed emotions had held me captive.

And maybe you've done something similar. Maybe, like me, you are a shining example of what I call a "good baby". If so, you are quite skilled at not expressing your emotions, at carting them around in a "contents under pressure" tank and thinking you are keeping the world a safer place by doing so.

Have you ever heard a baby who rarely cries called a "good baby"? This kind of comment consistently amazes me, because it indicates that from birth we are labeled as "good" based on our lack of emotional expression. And those of us who are quick learners soon realize this association between our lack of emotion and our perceived value as human beings.

There are cultural variations in this model, of course. Certain emotions are deemed suitable for expression by girls (grief, for instance), while others are considered more appropriate for boys to convey (such as anger). And natives of some regions seem to be more comfortable expressing their emotions than are people in other areas.

However, those of us currently living in the western world have certainly experienced the repression of emotions ~ if not our own, then those of others. You may have received a cutting remark from a store clerk and thought, "Wow, he is angry at something, but it surely isn't me!" Or maybe you've been around someone who cries buckets of tears over something that seems to you to be not exactly the full source of the person's grief.

Perhaps, like me, you learned a very powerful lesson at a young age: Only poorly behaved people or unstable people express their emotions, the rest of us rise above them and would never consider taking up any space with our own emotional responses to anything. I got very good at hiding my emotions ~ so good that at some point during my teenage years, I could no longer even identify my emotions; I just knew that they were bad and needed to be pushed aside.

But we all know that it is impossible to push emotions aside forever; they will someday surface, often in very harmful ways. These emotional outbursts all happen because most of us are like little time bombs, filled to overflowing with emotions we have refused to express and have instead locked away. We have clamped down on our anger, our grief, even our joy, because we are trying to be just like the "good" little babies who do not upset anyone around them with their emotions. The only problem with what we have done is that there is no "away". Just like trash hauled to a landfill, our emotions do indeed go somewhere when we do not express them.

Where they go is inside our very beings (where they can infest the cells of our physical bodies, the beliefs of our mental bodies, and the spiritual stores of our energetic bodies). These are the large tanks I see us each hauling around whose contents should be marked "under pressure". When someone or something happens to bump into our tank, we can release a huge amount of this dangerous substance that has been building and building over the years. It is dangerous not in its original source ~ which is just pure emotion; rather, it is dangerous, because it has been stored under pressure for so long.

When we do not release our emotions as we experience them, we add them to the ever-growing reservoirs already stored in us; and we become like walking, talking volcanoes, ready to explode our toxic waste all over the place.

It was only through giving birth to and raising two babies of my own that I began to learn this lesson. When they were small, my children did exactly what all small children do when they felt sad or angry or joyful ~ they expressed that! It was beautiful to watch, and it all seemed so simple: feel sad, express sadness, move on; feel angry, express anger, move on.

Even though I could appreciate the fluidity with which they expressed their emotions, I still was not able to emulate them quite yet. And they quickly learned this. When the kids were old enough to articulate their experiences, they began to ask questions like, "Are you mad at me?" or "Why is Daddy so sad?" I was so confused when I pondered these questions, because I couldn't find any words we had spoken or actions we had taken that would lead them to feel this way. Yet I still had the strong feeling that they were stating their truth; there was absolutely no manipulation or confusion on their part. It finally struck me that the children were more in touch with our emotions than we were. Their father and I had both become so accustomed to clenching our jaws and saying, "No, I'm not angry," or putting on a happy face and saying some sweet phrase in the midst of feeling really sad that we had no idea we were suppressing our emotions. Indeed, we often did not even realize we were feeling anything at all.

WOW! A brand new world opened up to me at that point! I realized that I hadn't been fooling anyone but myself with all this hiding of my emotions. And, in fact, I had not fooled myself really, because the hidden emotions always have a way of surfacing, if not in our emotional bodies then certainly in the physical or mental realms of our being.

Ironically, we often think we are keeping ourselves and our loved ones safe when we store our emotions rather than express them. The truth is, I feel about emotions the same way the lovable ogre Shrek feels about belches, "Better out than in, I always say!"

The element of Water is associated with our Emotional bodies, and its fluidity can be our guide as we work toward our emotional healing. Water can be as small as a tiny teardrop or as vast as the ocean, as slowly moving as a lazy river or as swift as a powerful waterfall. No matter what form it takes, though, water flows and moves; and our emotions flow and move the same way. They arise and they fall away.

But, just like water, emotions can be dammed up; and those dams we create throughout the years invariably break in messy, often painful ways. I picture repressed emotions going into a huge pot that sits quietly on a stove somewhere, simmering away. We keep adding to that pot and slowly turning the heat up under it, until the lid blows off in a burst of steam. We have taken our emotions, which are as pure and clean as fresh rainwater, and by ignoring them and stuffing them and adding stories to them, we have turned them into hot vapor that has the potential to burn all of those around us.

As we turn to the Emotional Body during this Spring Renewal, I invite you to take the lids off any emotional pots you may have simmering. It is helpful to approach our Emotional Spring Renewal from two different angles: 1. honoring our current emotions as they arise and 2. expressing any emotions we have stored away in our beings during our lifetimes. The first of these processes will help us approach the second.

This week, consider closely your emotional responses to different situations; simply work to recognize emotions as soon as they arise and to express them. Use a toddler as your guru here. When you feel sad, cry; when you feel angry, have a little tantrum; and when you feel joy, laugh and dance and shout.

Try to be present with your emotions as they arise and are expressed, and witness any reactions you have to this process. Your mind might have some opinions about this! That's okay; just repeatedly inform your mind that it can take a vacation during this exercise, because it has no business interfering with your emotions.

During the course of the week, you will likely find yourself in a situation when the emotions you are presently experiencing and expressing seem to be somehow linked to a larger well of emotions deep within you. That's great; you have found one of your pots! This is the perfect opportunity to begin releasing them before they turn into that scorching steam.

Sometimes our emotions are so deeply hidden that they may take some excavating to reach. We may realize, for instance, that we have a deep sadness somewhere, but we are not sure about the genesis of that grief. Fortunately, we do not always need to know its source in order to express it. We need to simply drill down beneath the surface and provide it with a channel through which to move. In fact, when we do not have a story related to an emotion, it is usually much easier to move that emotion.

Need help expressing something? A brilliant tool may be no further than your living room. I love to use films to help with my emotional expression. Who hasn't felt the relief of a "good cry" precipitated by watching some sappy scene in a movie? I recently realized that I have a whole stockroom of joy stored away in me that I was too afraid to ever express as a child, so my current work in this realm involves laughing until my sides hurt while viewing silly comedies. Use whatever stimulus you like to help pop the lid off your emotional reservoir, then allow those emotions to flow up and out of you.

Many blessings to each of us as we honor and express ourselves during this healing and renewal of our relationship with our emotional bodies. Let's get a little wet!!

Heart Healing Practices for the Emotional Body

Altar: Create an altar to healing and renewing the relationship with your emotional body. Incorporate any objects that you associate with this healing and renewal, including symbols of the element of Water. Spend time with your altar, connecting with your intent for healing and renewal.

Nature as Teacher: Dedicate some time to communing with the element of Water. Be open to any gifts of wisdom you may be given and integrate these into your healing and renewing of the relationship with your emotional body.

Sitting Practice: Breathe deeply into your heart. Begin to witness your emotional body. Without judgment or a need to change or shift anything, simply notice what is happening with your emotions. Observe if they seem to originate from or persist in specific areas of your physical body. Imagine that you can watch each one rise and fall away, much like the waves of the ocean. Next, direct energy from your heart outward to any places where emotions may be present, adding your own love to whatever form your emotions take.

Staying Current: Make it a practice to stay current with your emotions. As emotions arise throughout your day, simply allow them to move up and out of you.

Media Inspiration: When you find it difficult to release emotions ~ either current emotions or those that are in your "tank" ~ use movies, television shows, or works of literature to help stimulate your own emotions ~ and then let them flow.

Temple or Wonderland?
Spring Renewal of the Physical Body, Part I

Do you not know that your body is a temple of the Holy Spirit?
~ 1 Corinthians 6:19

Your body is a wonderland,
Your body is a wonder
~ John Mayer

What in the world could these two views of the human body have in common? The first, written by a perhaps overly zealous convert to Christianity, forms part of an admonition against "desires of the flesh," while the second is taken from a contemporary song of praise for a lover's body (very much related to those exact desires of the flesh being admonished in the modern melody). To me, they function as the perfect endpoints on a very long spectrum of ways we can view and treat our bodies. I also believe that they can be blended together to form a new way to treat our bodies ~ a healthy, respectful, and joyful way; but more about that soon . . . first let's consider them as opposites.

In our culture, we tend to approach our physical bodies from one of two extreme positions ~ either one of rigidity, strict boundaries, and an ill-conceived idea of "purity," or one of a carefree, party-until-dawn kind of gluttony. One quick review of magazines on the newsstands shows us that there are multiple ways in which we should be eating and exercising as well as a plethora of indulgences being offered to us. I particularly enjoy the magazine issues that follow detailed articles on new diet plans with pages of advertisements for sweet treats to purchase on our next supermarket run! Many of us swing back and forth between these two extremes, alternating between strict adherence to rules of denial, even punishment, and playing the role of rebellious teenager, by allowing ourselves to partake in every physical indulgence that comes our way. Some of us even play both the warden and the jail-breaker roles several times in the same day. Paul's letter and Mayer's song can serve as anthems for both extremes.

I see large-scale cultural evidence of these extreme models of body treatment in all manner of places. When we hear news of a new potentially deadly virus being found somewhere on the planet, many people respond with fear-based reliance on antidotes (which we often eventually learn will do more harm than good) and others show their lack of fear through possibly dangerous behaviors that make light of the situation. Some people respond to dietary and exercise guidelines by severely limiting what foods they eat and devising boot-camp-like regiments for fitness, and others choose to ignore this information and continue to eat and behave in ways we know may be unhealthy. Cravings are usually approached as things either to be totally indulged or strictly denied. It is as if each of us (or our cultural groups) has Paul on one shoulder repeating the temple bit and Mayer on the other singing about wonderlands. And we can (and do!) get confused.

But maybe the confusion lies in the idea that these concepts are opposites and that we must choose only one of them as a guide for how to treat our bodies.

Neither of these approaches is very healthy; both lead to extreme discomfort, pain, judgment, self-loathing, and often eventually disease. I believe that this is due in large part to us misunderstanding that our bodies are, indeed, both temples and wonderlands . . . and that there really is no difference between the two.

Upon first glance, many people in our society may say that our bodies cannot be both temples to God and wonderlands, that these two aspects of our physical being are mutually exclusive of one another. What do temples and wonderlands have to do with one another ~ specifically as they relate to our bodies? Is it blasphemous to even consider them together?

The New Testament quote has been used to instill

all kinds of worries and fears in people about their bodies. As we envision certain places of worship where we may have spent a good portion of time but where we have never felt quite at home, we ask, "If my body is a temple, then that means it has to be like some kind of church or synagogue, right?"

Yes and no.

Yes, our bodies are temples, in that they are infused with the Divine.

But no ~ they are not like churches . . . at least not the kinds with which many of us are familiar. To many people, temples, synagogues, mosques, and churches are buildings that seem austere, even scary. They are places to be visited only when in our most serene, most peaceful, most enlightened states; they are structures that house a kind of God that may feel very remote and removed from our own lives. And the New Testament verse comparing our bodies to temples is often used as evidence when people are admonished to treat their bodies as though they were holy ~ with a very limiting definition of what constitutes "holy".

However, I believe that to use the words in Paul's letter as fear-instilling dogmatic directions for holiness is to be reading them only from one viewpoint, one that is very narrow. I am much less concerned here with what Paul *meant* to convey with his words than I am with what may have actually been conveyed to the people to whom they were directed. To me, the former way of approaching the text is too limiting and, quite frankly, not very fruitful; messages may not ever have their exact intended effect, but they have an effect nonetheless. So, while Paul may have been traveling the countryside of Greece and teaching its inhabitants his very specific formula for holiness, those same inhabitants would be listening with ears, minds, and hearts ready to receive this information in a multitude of ways. We also have our own ears, minds, and hearts to receive messages, perhaps as they were intended, perhaps not.

Paul's letter was written to the Corinthians, people living in ancient Greece, and the word "temple" to them had a very specific meaning. A temple was the physical home of a god or goddess; it was a stone structure erected to both house the physical representation of the deity and to be a location where worshippers could honor that deity. However, a temple was in no way viewed as separate from daily life, an austere structure to be visited only once a week and where only very calm, serene, and respectful kinds of activities occurred. Greeks built temples in all different kinds of locations, from wild, rural vistas to the centers of towns; and these locations were determined by the specific aspects of the specific deity being worshipped. For instance, Athena's presence was felt, observed, and worshipped on the Athenian Acropolis long before any temples were erected to honor it. Temples were permanent constructions built to physically define space as sacred, but the space was already sacred. In other words, the divine was already present, the worship and honor were already being done; the temple just provided a physical location for that connection between worshiper and deity.

And I see our bodies as functioning pretty much in the same way ~ the divine exists everywhere and always. I just get to use this body in this lifetime as a physical location to house the divine and with which to worship the divine. Many people also view our physical bodies in this light; where we may differ, though, is in what we consider to be "worship" and in how we approach the care-taking of these temples.

Here again, I like to consider that Paul's words were specifically directed at the Greeks, and the Greeks worshiped the divine in a multitude of ways ~ some of which may seem startling to those of us who were raised within contemporary Western religious traditions. Greek rituals could take the form of healing dreaming ceremonies, of drinking festivals, of dramatic plays, of athletic competitions, of bawdy women-only nights held to teach adolescent girls about their bodies; indeed, they could take almost any form imaginable, because to the ancient Greeks there was no distinction between what was holy and what was not. They went to their temples and sanctuaries to sell things, to meet with people, to have feasts . . . and all of this was considered worship. If this sounds strange to you, you might consider the craft bazaars and potluck dinners held at many large places of worship today.

These temples sound pretty much like wonderlands, don't they?

Our bodies also, are, wonderlands ~ places of healing, dreaming, revelry, play, movement, bawdiness, and so much more. And we are the guardians, protectors, stewards, and revelers of these wonderlands. We would do very well to keep them clean. But just how do we do that? How do we take care of these wonderland temples without using either extreme of harsh denial or overindulgence?

We do this by each finding our own perfect balance, and for me the ideal teacher of this lesson is Gaia, Mother Earth.

I invite you to spend some time observing two different divine bodies: yours and that of the Earth. Pay attention to places of balance in each, to places of imbalance; to ways in which each are cleansed, nourished, and enjoyed.

Heart Healing Practices for your Temple-Wonderland

Altar: Create an altar to healing and renewing the relationship with your physical body. Incorporate any objects that you associate with this healing and renewal, including symbols of the element of Earth. Spend time with your altar, connecting with your intent for healing and renewal.

Nature as Teacher: Dedicate some time to communing with the element of Earth. Be open to any gifts of wisdom you may be given and integrate these into your healing and renewing of the relationship with your physical body; in particular, you may pay attention to things in nature that are sacred and joyful to you.

Sitting Practice: Breathe deeply into your heart. Scan your physical form, observing what is happening in your body in this moment. Next, send energy from your heart outward to your entire body, offering gratitude for this amazing Temple-Wonderland.

Temple-Wonderland Consecration: Create a ritual to honor your physical form. You may choose to use as inspiration any ceremonies used to show respect to sacred buildings or sites ~ or anything else that helps you celebrate your unique Temple-Wonderland!

Find Your Perfect Balance: Spring Renewal of the Physical Body, Part II

Of the four elements, Earth is the densest form of matter; it is the only solid of the elements. Similarly, our Physical Beings are our aspects with the most density. They have weight, mass, and volume, and this means that they may show signs of change more slowly than do the other realms of our being. In this modern world, where things can happen so quickly ~ communications are sent across the globe in mere seconds, meals can be made in minutes ~ many of us want to see immediate evidence of what we are doing with our bodies. We want healing to happen in the blink of an eye, and we want dietary changes and new exercise routines to show results instantly. Sometimes the quick changes do happen. And sometimes, change may only appear in our bodies, as it does in the earth, over time. In this way, Mother Earth can teach us the importance of patience when dealing with our physical beings.

Just as our bodies appear to change more slowly than do other aspects of our being (our thoughts can shift quickly, for instance, and emotions arise within seconds), our *relationships* with our physical form often change over time rather than immediately. Indeed, our physical bodies are the first aspects of our being with which we develop relationships; as babies begin to experience themselves as separate from other beings around them, it is their bodies that are the first form of distinction. They realize that their forms are "theirs" long before they can conceptualize their individual minds, emotions, or spirits.

So your relationship with your body is among the earliest of relationships we experience in this lifetime. You may have long and deeply-entrenched patterns of relating with your body. And shifting those can take time and may involve a multi-layered approach that benefits from much patience.

And yet, at the microcosmic level, physical bodies do change incredibly rapidly. Our skin regenerates all the time, for instance, and our cells divide and multiply at a phenomenal rate. So, just like with the Earth, while changes may not be obviously visible right away, they are happening continually. In this way, the element of Earth provides us with lessons of adaptability in our bodies as wells as acceptance of change.

Whether modifications happen gradually or instantaneously, they do happen ~ both in the planet where we reside and in the bodies in which we reside. I have found that for me to accept and embrace these changes most easily, I need to consistently create balance within my physical being, and this is yet another area where I use the

Earth as a teacher.

Mother Earth is always seeking and finding balance. Sometimes this balance comes through the juxtaposition of extremes (years of drought followed by a huge flood, for instance) and other times the balance takes a more subtle form. Our bodies seem to me to always be searching for balance, and healing and renewing our relationship with my physical body involves finding and celebrating that sense of balance in my body.

How do we bring the lessons from earth into our Physical Spring Renewal? We have been gifted with these beautiful, magical bodies ~ these temple wonderlands. How do we go about healing them, without the harsh chemicals of judgment and rigidity and the madness of overindulgence? For me, the trick lies in paying attention not only to *what* I am doing to my body but to *how* I am doing it; it involves finding what is truly good for me and what substances are toxic to my body, mind, and spirit.

I once attended a lovely spiritual retreat with my family and many friends, where we were blessed to eat delicious, wholesome food prepared by a talented chef. One day, I walked into the kitchen and heard one of the adults lecturing the children about the importance of eating an organic, vegetarian diet. She went on and on about the dangers of ingesting pesticides along with our fruits and vegetables and about eating hormones along with our beef. I watched the kids lose energy and gain fear with each sentence, with each terrifying fact presented to them about what harm may have already been done to their young bodies. I suddenly thought, "Are they not also being fed the poison of fear right now?"

I, too, have been fed that very same poison, and I have felt its affects on my body. I once attended a lecture given by a holistic dentist, where I learned a multitude of things about what horrible elements had been used in dentistry in previous decades. However, rather than using this information to fuel a change in my dental care, I simply took in what was really being communicated to me ~ fear. "What in the world is in my mouth?" I thought, "Am I a time-bomb of mercury just waiting to turn into physical and psychological disease?" The information itself was very good; it was the *manner* in which it was presented and the way in which I received it that made the situation feel toxic.

Examples of important information about health being presented and received in unhealthy ways abound. A few years ago, much of the western world was gripped in fear about the swine flu "epidemic". Entire school systems closed, people avoided travel, and everywhere I looked I saw enormous bottles of antibacterial gel being wielded like weapons against this dangerous invader. And it was a *very* serious situation . . . for a *very* small number of people. As someone who lives with a chronic health condition and a compromised immune system, I do pay attention to such situations and I take what I feel are the appropriate and necessary precautions for myself. However, I do not imprison myself and my family in our home and listen to the never-ending news reports detailing just how large the danger is.

I appreciate that many people respond well to the kind of fear-infused messages found in the media. I do not. I just take in the fear. How is that helpful? Isn't that poison too? So, I have found that I must be diligent about separating out the information from the poison with which it is so easily infected.

We have all learned, for instance, that overuse of antibiotics and even antibacterial cleaners can be every bit as harmful as are the diseases we are attempting to avoid by using them. So . . . do we need to stay away from them entirely? There are many people who would suggest that we do; however, there are millions of lives that have been saved by antibiotics since their momentous discovery.

We are blessed to live in a time when we have great access to information about our bodies and how to take care of them; however, it sometimes feels as though I have *too much* information in this area. I can read evidence that supports the strengths of a diet rich in whole-grain foods immediately after I review evidence that indicates that grains should be avoided altogether. There are any number of experts who promote excluding all foods that are derived from animal sources . . . and many who now argue that we should be eating meat and excluding legumes. And yes, each of them is correct: a raw, vegan diet works beautifully with some bodies; a "paleo" diet seems most appropriate for others; and there are still ~ as difficult as this may seem to believe ~ people living who thrive on healthy sources of whole grains and dairy products. And what is best for any individual body during one particular period of life may not be best a few years later.

So, how do we know what is right for our particular body? How do we find the perfect balance for us? We listen, first and foremost, to our bodies. With every new bit of "evidence" we receive from "experts," we must first check in with the only real expert about our body ~ us! Our bodies *can* and *do* tell us exactly what they need; it just may take a bit of work for us to be able to hear them and to decipher the messages being sent.

One tool I love to use in this process of Spring Renewal is a dietary cleanse. I use these cleanses as a way of resetting my system. Once I have gotten rid of substances that are not my body's best fuel sources and after I have broken any habits that may involve such substances, I can clearly receive the messages my body sends me. There are any number of cleanses that one can do, from 40-day-liquid-only cleanses to day-long fasts to just eating fruits and veggies for a few days. We each need to find the ones that work best to reset our bodies to neutral, so that we can get clear information from them.

I invite you to do a little dietary cleanse of your own, to get your body back to neutral. This may involve letting go of your Diet Coke habit for a few days, or it may mean introducing a new fruit or vegetable into your diet each day for a week. We can get some very useful information about our temples this way!

I also encourage you to really pay attention to the information you take in regarding your body and how to best care for it; maybe it is time to cleanse some of that as well? Hopefully, we can wash out some of the negativity and fear that imbue so much of the "helpful hints" we are continually receiving, ridding our beings of that type of poison as well.

However you choose to heal and renew your relationship with your physical body, I support you in doing it with love, compassion, and a sense of balance.

Heart Healing Practices for Body Balance

Altar: Create an altar to healing and renewing the relationship with your physical body. Incorporate any objects that you associate with this healing and renewal, including symbols of the element of Earth. Spend time with your altar, connecting with your intent for healing and renewal.

Nature as Teacher: Dedicate some time to communing with the element of Earth. Be open to any gifts of wisdom you may be given and integrate these into your healing and renewing of the relationship with your physical body; in particular, you may pay attention to ways the Earth seeks and creates Balance.

Sitting Practice: Breathe deeply into your heart. Scan your physical form, observing what is happening in your body in this moment. Next, watch your mind's reaction to your physical form. What thoughts arise when you contemplate your body? Simply observe any judgments, any "poison" thoughts, and direct energy from your heart to your mind as these forms. Imagine your own essence bathing your mind, washing away the poison of judgment and replacing it with love.

Cleanse: Spend some time ~ an hour, a day, a week ~ engaged in either a dietary cleanse or a thought-cleanse. Ask your body itself what type of cleanse it would like, rather than turning to information from other sources. If you choose to perform a thought-cleanse, dedicate yourself to purging any negative body-thoughts; as they arise, imagine them being flushed out of your system and replaced with healing, cleansing body-thoughts.

True Nourishment: Spring Renewal of the Physical Body, Part III

We each get just one of these precious bodies, these wonderland temples, for this entire lifetime; yet, we often do not treat them like we would any other cherished one-of-a-kind treasure. We deny them exercise and rest and play and love; we sometimes forget about their true nourishment entirely, yet we expect them to keep performing in top form at all times.

We often go for days, weeks (some of us even go for years) without really considering our bodies' needs in terms of nutrition, exercise, and rest. If we treated our cars the way we often treat our bodies, we would drive them endlessly, even recklessly, on the cheapest gas available and only take them to be serviced when they had broken down.

It is vital that we shift the way we nourish our bodies; yet, so many of us do that harshly rather than lovingly. We may decide to "care for" our physical beings by becoming little drill sergeants whose job it is to "whip them into shape" with stringent exercise routines and restrictive diets based on the recommendations of everyone around us. That surely isn't the way we would treat a temple, is it? And the results of such an approach often do not look or feel anything like a wonderland.

Why consult with all those external sources of information about our bodies, when the real experts are right here at hand ~ and foot and head and everywhere in between? Our bodies repeatedly tell us how to nourish them, to provide what they need in order for them to continue serving as the sacred containers of our beautiful souls.

Each of us knows how to do this. Our bodies know what they need; it may just take awhile for the rest of us to remember. Like all other living organisms, we have an innate ability to seek the things that nourish us; and when I need to be reminded of this wonderful fact of nature, I need only to look outside of my window.

Living in south Texas for several years provided me with numerous lessons about how life can thrive, even in the harshest of conditions. After a period of steady rain for a full year, the area entered into a severe drought that persisted for two full years. During this time, the earth was parched, crops withered, farm animals became emaciated, and gardeners sometimes had difficulty getting anything to pop up out of the ground. Spring in this region can bring a bounty of wildflowers that color the fields everywhere; but not one year in particular during my time there ~ that year, even the treasured bluebonnets were nowhere to be seen.

This following fall, though, the rains returned ~

steady, consistent rains that reached deep into the soil to nourish the roots struggling to take hold there. After so many months of dryness, it often takes the earth a bit of time to be able to soak in the fresh waters; but the ground eventually softens and takes in the nutrients raining down from the heavens.

We may feel as though our physical beings are much like the drought-ridden south Texas soil, parched and cracked. But, just as the earth remembers how to accept the rains, our bodies can remember how to receive the nurturing flow of healthy food, exercise, and rest. Bit by bit, we can learn to soak in the love of physical nurturing.

One of the ways our bodies communicate their needs with us is through cravings; however, this is a type of message that many of us either ignore or misunderstand, and that is because we may be confused about what a true craving really is. Our habitual behaviors may create feelings of want or desire (sometimes even of need) that are not *true* cravings. For instance, if I have a pattern of drinking a large iced mocha with lots of chocolate each afternoon, my body will get used to that, and I may soon discover that I feel very different if I skip this treat one day. My body will certainly crave the sugar and caffeine it is used to and is now being denied, but this is not necessarily a healthy craving.

We can also have cravings that *feel* like physical cravings but that originate not in our physical bodies at all; instead, they may be emotional or mental cravings that masquerade as physical needs. If I find I have the urge for tomato sauce and melted mozzarella only when I smell a pizza, then the urge is not physical. Likewise, if I suddenly feel a desire for a glass of wine when I see someone else drinking one, then that is not a physical desire. If I find myself wanting chocolate chip cookies directly after having my feelings hurt, then I am probably having an emotional craving (for comfort, let's say) rather than a physical one.

True cravings can be incredibly powerful tools for use in our bodies' nourishment. Pregnant women frequently crave the very foods they need to sustain their bodies during the intense changes they are experiencing, just as we often desire to refrain from eating when it would harm our bodies to do so. The trick for me is to listen to what my body tells me it needs rather than what my mind or my emotions may be saying. And then to always honor that by providing my physical being with the nutrients it craves.

Similarly, our bodies send us many messages about how they would like to be moved and exercised ~ messages we often ignore, if we receive them at all. I am blessed with a body that has drastically variable exercise capacities. I can walk for an hour one day and then have difficulty climbing the stairs the following day. So I get to listen ~ and respond. Again, I must really listen to my body in order to receive the true message being sent. My mind is not helpful here, as it may tell me things like, "Oh, it is cold outside; I really don't feel well enough to walk today," or "I just did this yesterday, I'm sure I can do it again today. I WILL do it again today."

I have learned to be very careful when I feel myself using judgment to "encourage" my body to exercise or to do anything in particular. I recently had planned to go to an evening yoga class, because my children's spring break interfered with my usual morning practice routine. Sitting with my family, I had the thought, "I don't want to be away from home tonight." Was that good information for me? Was it that I really needed to stay home, since I'd been away for the previous five nights? Was I being lazy by not going to yoga? Was I letting myself down by not fulfilling an obligation I had made to myself? My daughter said, "I have an idea. Why don't you do yoga at home?" Indeed, why not? So I did what I have to do in order to get in touch with my body's truest needs and desires: I got very quiet and listened to all the information coming in ~ from my body, from my mind, from my Spirit. And I was given the perfect answer! My body wanted to both move and be with my family. So, my partner and I loaded the children, their bikes, and a yoga mat into the car and drove to a nearby high school, where the kids rode bikes and played football with their father while I did my practice in the fresh spring air. And, as a huge bonus, I rode a bicycle for the first time in over ten years!! If I had listened to the critic in my head and attended the yoga class simply because I was following my own rules, I would have missed that opportunity.

Just like with food and exercise, our bodies know exactly how much rest they need; we just need to listen to them and give them the rest for which they are begging us! I am blessed with a body that needs physical rest more often than it used to. Before my heart and lungs became compromised, I rarely sat down. I spent years in academia, teaching and working in museums and studying ~ and resting very, very little. I would finally fall into bed late at night and awaken very early the next morning to begin running around all over again.

When my first child was born, I was so used to running around that I had to really work to make myself sit still for any length of time. But watching him grow and nurturing him taught me something ~ I needed to rest every bit as much as this little infant did. He was a big baby who nursed every two hours for hour-long stretches. Sitting still for this amount of time was difficult for me to do at first, so I created assignments to do while feeding him (bills to pay, phone calls to make, etc). But his restlessness during those times when I was multi-tasking taught me to slow down and focus on what was happening: I was nurturing and nourishing another human being. How could there be anything more important than that? I learned to really rest into the time and space where I was, to be present for myself and my son and to enjoy this precious time with him. I knew that I used to be able to do just that ~ to rest, to be present ~ when I was a child; I had simply forgotten how to do that as an adult.

When I became ill soon after that, I found that I benefitted greatly from a short nap time each afternoon. I would lie down for 20-30 minutes, sometimes to sleep, sometimes not ~ but always to dream. During these periods, so many beautiful gifts have been given to me in dreams and visions. I am not only elevating my feet and resting my heart and lungs, I am nourishing my mind and my spirit. So I find that I am quite fortunate that I get to have my "dreamtime" most afternoons. And I often wonder how I ever lived without this vital part of my life. Even those of us who need fewer hours of sleep than others may not need fewer hours of *rest*.

My kids taught me the beauty of listening to their bodies. When they are tired, they rest. That makes perfect sense and seems so obvious, yet why don't we all do that?

Because we have simply forgotten, that's all.

But we can remember. Our bodies can remember what is nourishing and good and healthy, even if the last time we were providing them with these things is when we were infants drinking breast milk, sleeping as much as we needed, releasing our emotions as they arose, and taking lots of time for wonder and play.

And just like that parched south Texas earth, our bodies are waiting for the nurturing that they need. This spring following a winter rich with moisture will produce, an area awash in wildflowers ~ the exquisite result of the soil taking in that long-absent rainwater. And when we remember those things that truly nourish us ~ good food, enjoyable exercise, and peaceful rest ~ and shower our beautiful bodies with them, we also flourish as the exquisite wildflowers we are.

Heart Healing Practices for True Nourishment

Altar: Create an altar to healing and renewing the relationship with your physical body. Incorporate any objects that you associate with this healing and renewal, including symbols of the element of Earth. Spend time with your altar, connecting with your intent for healing and renewal.

Nature as Teacher: Dedicate some time to communing with the element of Earth. Be open to any gifts of wisdom you may be given and integrate these into your healing and renewing of the relationship with your physical body; in particular, you may pay attention to examples of True Nourishment that exist in nature.

Sitting Practice: Breathe deeply into your heart. Scan your physical form, observing what is happening in your body in this moment. Next, ask your body what it needs right now in terms of nourishment, movement, and rest. After each question, wait for your body's true response to arise. It may take almost any form, such as words, an image, a memory, a feeling, an emotion. Honor your body's request by committing to provide it with the nourishment, movement, and rest it needs.

True Nourishment: For one day, feed your body exactly what it requests. Listen to it carefully to determine if the request is coming from a true physical need or an emotional, mental, or energetic craving. Another day, give your body all the movement it requests (again, carefully watching for any thought-based or emotion-fueled desires). On yet another day, provide your body with all the rest it craves, judgment-free.

EnJOYing our Bodies: Spring Renewal of the Physical Body, Part IV

Do you enjoy yourself while swimming in public places?

Can you have fun when you know that other people are seeing you in your swimsuit?

I recently asked two friends these questions, and I received two very different answers. Friend A said, "No, I rarely wear a swimsuit in public, and if I do I am worried about how I look the entire time. I never even focus on having fun."

And Friend B said, "Absolutely! If the suit fits me, I put it on and forget about it; and I have a great time!"

Obviously one of these women experiences joy in her physical body when swimming in public, and the other woman is unable to do so. This is not so surprising; we know that many people (particularly women) feel uncomfortable wearing clothing that reveals their physical forms. What may be surprising, though, is that Friend A, the woman who did not enjoy such experiences, fits perfectly within the standards that our culture has set for what an attractive woman is. She is young, thin, and fit. Friend B, on the other hand, is very heavy; indeed, she has a difficult time finding bathing suits to fit her large frame.

How did that happen? How does a young woman

who would look absolutely at home in the swimsuit edition of Sports Illustrated *not* feel good about her body? How does a woman whose obesity is actually a health concern feel *good* about her body? And how in the world can the rest of us learn to feel good about our bodies as well?

These are not new questions to me. In fact, I've been asking them ever since I was a teenager and began to really pay attention to the complicated relationship many people (particularly women) raised in contemporary Western culture have with their bodies.

I moved to Greece when I was sixteen, and upon my arrival I was immediately invited to go to the beach with some kids my age. I was thrilled with the invitation and so excited to actually immerse my body in the brilliant blue waters of the Mediterranean Sea. Yet worries followed right on the heels of my excitement ~ worries that my swimsuit wasn't cute enough, that my tan wasn't dark enough, that my body wasn't fit enough ~ in general, that *I* wasn't "enough" to be able to be at the beach, that my body was somehow not as deserving of the experience as were the bodies of my peers.

The "evidence" to support this belief ~ that some bodies deserve experiences more than others, simply because they look a certain way ~ is all around me still. Every time I see magazine pictures of celebrities that are accompanied by captions like "Stars with Cellulite" and "Back in Shape Two Seconds After Giving Birth to Twins", I am reminded that swimming trips and beach adventures can be turned into occasions for scrutiny and ridicule . . . even for those of us who are not celebrities. I am always amazed by some comments I hear when I go to swimming pools and water parks, comments about the bodies of others there, comments like, "Wow, she really shouldn't be seen in public like that." And I always think, "Why not?" Such comments imply that only people who look a certain way should have the opportunity to feel the warmth of the sun on their skin and to enjoy cooling off in the water.

And at sixteen years old, I had already learned that lesson well. That day, in the moment when my focus shifted from my excitement to my worries, all joy left my body. At that instant, my awareness was no longer on my own experience at all; rather, it was on what other people would think of me. I was not able to find enjoyment in my body, because I was no longer really in my body at all – I was over in everyone else's heads, trying to figure out what *they* thought about my body. I wasn't *feeling* my body at all; I was feeling something *about* my body, and there is an enormous difference between these two things.

It is absolutely impossible to enjoy our bodies, to find joy ~ or, rather, to create joy ~ in them, unless we are actually *in* them. Many of us continually rob ourselves of the opportunity to enjoy our bodies, and we do this exactly like I did as a teenager on the beach – we do not really inhabit them at all. So our work in learning to enjoy our bodies is to *be* in them, right here, right now. I know that may sound a little strange, and you may be thinking, "Of course I am in my body; where else would I be?" Let's see . . .

Are you currently feeling your body? Are you experiencing the affect of countless stimuli on each of your senses ~ without judging those sensations or even naming them? Or, like most of us most of the time, are you avoiding feeling something in your body or attempting to feel something different in your body? Are you labeling sounds and smells around you as good or bad; are you trying to create new sounds and smells or get away from others?

Although each of us is blessed to be in a human body during this lifetime, we may not spend very much time actually being in that body. We may spend more time in our minds or in our emotional bodies, and we certainly spend a lot of time in our bodies as they *used to be* (through memories) and our bodies as we *wish* they were or are *planning* on them becoming (through fantasies).

We didn't always do this. We certainly did not do this when we were babies; have you ever watched babies enjoying their bodies? They do so absolutely and thoroughly, because they are absolutely and thoroughly present with their physical experiences. I remember when my children were infants and they discovered each of their body parts, one by one. The look of wonder and joy as babies move and experiment with their bodies is amazing; it is as though they are discovering a fascinating toy with each movement! Why don't adults experience the same wonder and fascination with their bodies?

The inability to do this happens over time, of course. By the time most of us are adults, our bodies are no longer toys, no longer wonderlands; instead, they often function as tools that we force to do whatever we like, they can play the role of big carrying cases for our brains and personalities, and they may even be sources of identity for us. In order to enjoy our bodies, in order to find enjoyment in them, we must change the way we experience our bodies. We must redirect our attention away from our thoughts and feelings and back to our bodies.

When we shift our attention back to our actual physical experiences, we can begin to feel the same joy that children feel. This process may involve retraining ourselves on several different levels. Fortunately, this training is very simple and always involves the same, exact method ~ coming back to right here, right now and simply experiencing our bodies. Simple; not at all easy.

The path to fully enjoying our bodies must involve us releasing all rules, regulations, and judgments about our bodies, about bodies in general. Many times when we want to enjoy our bodies, we do so with conditions ~ for example, we can enjoy our bodies once we look a certain way, we can enjoy our bodies only after all our "work" is done, we can enjoy sharing our bodies with others only within very limited and restricting societal rules about relationships.

Unfortunately, most of us have spent decades using such rules, regulations, and judgments in order to overcome our bodies, to get them to perform or look in specified ways; this means we need to consistently practice a new way of being with (being *in*) our bodies.

In this practice, we consistently bring our awareness back to the physical sensations we have right here, right now. When we find that we are exercising with goals of looking a specific way, or forcing our bodies to sit still for hours on end when they really want to move, or comparing our bodies with those of anyone else (even the bodies we used to have!), we simply note that we are using our old ways of interacting with our bodies ~ that we are having thoughts or beliefs about our bodies and have thus left our physical beings and jumped into our mental or emotional beings.

No problem; we can now redirect our focus back to

the physical sensations of our physical bodies.

Again . . . and again . . . and again . . .

My friend who allowed herself to enjoy swimming in public knew this trick. Her attention was on her body, not outside of it. She was experiencing her physical body, rather than thinking about it or having feelings about it.

My other friend was not able to do this. Her focus was outside of herself, on what other people thought of her; she therefore was identifying with thoughts or beliefs about her body.

This habit of identifying with thoughts (usually with what we assume to be others' thoughts about our bodies) can begin when we are children. We hear comments like, "Comb your hair; what will people think?" and "Surely you aren't going to wear *that* in public," and we receive the message that our comfort, our feeling good in our own skin, should always be considered secondary to our not offending others aesthetically. An astute child will often quickly learn to identify with his or her appearance, to identify with the way he or she looks. As soon as we do this, we are no longer able to fully inhabit our bodies, because we are now identifying with them as visual objects being viewed by others. And each time we alter our appearance (with haircuts, specific clothing, tattoos, or anything else) with any thought to what others may think or feel about us, we are identifying with *our* assumptions about *their* ideas about *our* bodies. WHEW! Where is the physical experience in *that*?

We are in bodies; yet, we are not our bodies, and we certainly are not the thoughts that other people have about our bodies ~ or what we think are the thoughts that other people may be having about our bodies. We layer thoughts and beliefs and assumptions on top of our physical experiences much like we layer our actual bodies with numerous layers of clothing to protect us from a huge snowstorm. No wonder many of us cannot enjoy the feeling of warm sun and cool water on our skin ~ we have so many layers covering up our physical sensations we may no longer even know that we *have* physical sensations.

Looking back to that day at the beach, I remember how surprised I was to realize that the rules I had learned in America about acceptable beach presentation did not apply in my new home. Naked babies were tended to by elderly grandpas wearing Speedos. I saw people of all ages and all sizes, wearing a huge variety of different attire. My "layers" of thoughts and judgment immediately evaporated, and I was then able to return to my real body, the one that exists always underneath those suffocating outer skins. And only then was I able to enjoy myself, to find joy in my body.

I still find that I've pulled some of those other skins back on, those layers that I use to protect myself but that actually insulate me from my true experiences, from my true joy. And, when I do, I return my attention to my body – right here, right now.

We are blessed with these physical forms for such a short time. Wouldn't it be nice to actually fully inhabit them, just like we did when we were babies? Wouldn't it be lovely to peel off those layers of insulating thoughts, judgments, and resentments with which we may be covering our physical beings so that we can feel the warmth of the sun on our skin?

Meet you at the beach . . .

Heart Healing Practices for Body EnJOYment

Altar: Create an altar to healing and renewing the relationship with your physical body. Incorporate any objects that you associate with this healing and renewal, including symbols of the element of Earth. Spend time with your altar, connecting with your intent for healing and renewal.

Nature as Teacher: Dedicate some time to communing with the element of Earth. Be open to any gifts of wisdom you may be given and integrate these into your healing and renewing of the relationship with your physical body; in particular, you may pay attention to all the things in nature that bring you enjoyment.

Sitting Practice: Sit outside in the sunshine; make yourself comfortable, close your eyes, and breathe deeply into your heart. Focus on one sense at a time, opening yourself up to fully engage with that sense ~ the sensations you feel on your skin and hair; the things you smell; the sounds around you; anything you may taste; and finally (gently opening your eyes) all the colors and forms your eye can see. End your practice by radiating love outward from your heart to your entire physical form, offering gratitude for your senses.

Peeling Back the Layers: For an entire day, track any thoughts you have about your physical appearance. Without judgment, simply write them down as they arise. At the end of the day, notice any repeating thoughts and any patterns. Imagine these thoughts layered upon you like bulky clothing. Picture yourself peeling off one thought-layer at a time, feeling your body relax more and more with each disappearing layer. Once all the "layers" have been removed, focus on breathing into your entire physical form, from the crown of your head to the tips of your toes, and offering gratitude for your amazing body.

Spring Renewal through Forgiveness

Clean Monday, the Greek holiday that ushers in the Lenten season, actually begins on the previous Sunday. Before all the festivities, before the cleaning and the kite flying and the picnicking, worshippers go to church for Forgiveness Vespers. During this ritual, each turns to the others and asks for forgiveness.

Why? What does this have to do with cleaning? How is forgiveness related to the preparation for new life that is celebrated throughout this season?

Forgiveness is perhaps the most important task that we can perform in healing and renewing our relationship with the different aspects of our being. Each of us carries with us places where we are still unable to forgive a person or a situation (or oftentimes ourselves), and those places act like clutter in our closets, clutter that may seem deceptively small but which takes up vast amounts of space in our lives.

There is a reason we refer to the lack of forgiveness as "holding a grudge;" because when we are not able to forgive we are actually grasping something. And, just as physically grasping something takes energy, this holding onto something does as well. We carry the places where we still need to forgive around with us like treasured belongings, and these treasures may show up in our physical bodies, in our energetic bodies, or in our emotional bodies.

I view the places where I have not yet forgiven someone or something as huge holes in my energetic field. I consistently lose energy through these holes; so even though I may continue to raise all the energy I can, if I have areas that are still unclean through lack of forgiveness, some of that new energy will just seep out of me.

Some of us may carry bits of clutter in our emotional bodies. If so, we will often continue to cycle stories around specific events and people, and this cycling makes us unable to release the emotions that need to flow forth. The result is that we are continually adding to our deep reservoirs of repressed emotions.

When our lack of forgiveness is stored in our physical bodies, it can manifest in any number of ailments, as we hoard this clutter in our cells, our tissue, our muscles, and our organs. Recent studies have found clear evidence that a patient's practice of forgiveness can greatly reduce the effects of some specific physical diseases, including high blood pressure, muscular tension, and chronic back pain.

Okay, so forgiveness can lead to more energy, greater emotional flow, and a healthier physical body. Let's play a little game to see if we can experience a bit of what that might actually *feel* like:

Close your eyes. Bring to mind someone or something that you have not yet forgiven. Hold the image of this person or situation in front of you and really, really focus on it. Now notice what your body has done: where are you holding this in your body, and how much energy is directed at that location?

Come back to a neutral state and take some deep breaths.

Now consciously bring that person or situation back into your awareness. But this time visualize them as though you have already forgiven them (this may mean recalling the feeling state of forgiving someone or something else and grafting it onto the person or situation in question). Now notice what your body has done.

What is the difference?

Which way do you *want* to feel?

We all want more of all that feeling, so we open up to the concept of forgiveness.

Now what? Sure, to "forgive and forget" seems sweet and simple and may be possible for others to do easily and continually; but what about the rest of us – how do *we* get there?

For me, learning to forgive has been a path ~ a spiritual path ~ that looked nothing like I would have expected. It took me years to actually begin to open to the possibility of forgiveness. And once I did open to the possibility, I still was not ready to forgive, because I was confused about what forgiveness actually *was*.

For years, I confused forgiveness with reconciliation. I thought that forgiving someone meant that I then needed to be in relationship with that person. That is not at all the case! Forgiveness and reconciliation are not same. And although forgiveness may be a prerequisite for reconciliation, the opposite is not true ~ reconciliation is not necessary for forgiveness.

That is because forgiveness really has nothing to do with the persons we are forgiving at all. They need not apologize; they need not feel sorry; they need not even know that we are forgiving them.

Forgiveness is about healing our own lives. We are vessels for the divine to shine through, and we clean our beings so that we may shine brightly. When we release those grudges we have been holding, we create more space in our lives ~ space for divine flow and inspiration and magic. Why wouldn't we choose to work toward that?

Another point of confusion for me was that I was trying to forgive or "get over it" from a place of attachment. By forgiving, I had to actually accept fully that something had happened, and that was very hard. When we choose to withhold forgiveness, we often do so because we are very attached to our concept of how things "should have been". When we choose to live without such judgments and attachments, forgiveness becomes more accessible to us.

I used to feel that if I forgave someone, I was somehow weak and that I was very tough and strong when I held firm in my lack of forgiveness. I think that I had the belief that if I forgave someone for something, I was opening myself up to having a similar thing happen again. If I forgive this person or this situation, I am somehow saying that what happened was okay, right? No; I am simply saying that what happened *happened*.

When we hold that belief that we are keeping ourselves safe by not forgiving, we are setting ourselves up in a ping-pong game of Judge and Victim, where we get to star in both leading roles. When I do not forgive, I can stand in judgment of the person or the situation that "wronged" me and I can get a tremendous amount of juice out of feeling sorry for myself for the ways in which this wronging was executed.

In the Judge-Victim matrix, blame rules everything, and blame seems to me to be self-indulgent (as does guilt, which is where we live when we cannot forgive ourselves for something). When I am in blame or in guilt, I am not actually able to take any action. When I am in blame, there is no space for forgiveness, for learning, for growth. Blame is all that can exist in that space, and it grows exponentially as I feed it attention. Self-blame that masquerades as awareness functions in this same way. As I notice some way in which I have been wronged by another or in which I have done something wrong, blame gets me stuck in a cycle so that I do not have to take any action, do not have to change things. It keeps the energy on the drama level, the story level, and out of the level of real movement, of real intent.

The models of forgiveness we are often given seem to me to be akin to a benevolent ruler bestowing forgiveness on someone, just as though she had waved a magic wand. So, is that how we forgive someone – we just wave some magic wand?

Believe me ~ I tried that, but it never worked! I kept waving that wand and repeating the mantra, "I forgive; all is forgiven," and waiting and waiting to feel something. But forgiveness is not a feeling! We may get to a feeling at some point ~ or perhaps the lack of a feeling ~ but forgiveness is an action, a practice. And for me, it was like my other spiritual practices. It took time and devotion and sometimes looked pretty darn messy. And, just like with those practices, I found one day that I could do it! And then I might pop out, just like I do in meditation or a yoga posture. So, I get back to the practice.

For me, that practice involves several steps, each of which can be related to different parts of my being:

1. Emotional release: I allow my emotions surrounding the event or person to flow freely, without attaching any stories to them.

2. Mental clarity without judgment: I work to fully accept the situation has happened. If I find I have attachments to how things "should have" been or how someone "should have" behaved, I have to unravel those to find their underlying assumptions and beliefs.

3. Physical cleansing: I try to locate any places in my body where I might be holding this grudge, and I continually visualize those places being purified by the flow of love from my heart chakra.

4. Energetic reclamation: I work to reclaim the energy I have lost through the situation or event and my holding onto it, by imagining holes in my energy being filled in and my entire field shining the pure bright light of love that I am.

Sometimes, the spiritual practice of forgiveness comes quite easily, and there have been situations and people it has taken me great amounts of time, focus, and energy to forgive and release. We just have a firmer grasp on some of these "treasures" we are carrying than others, and our fingers may take a bit of prying to enable us to finally put down these loads. And that can be difficult.

The results, however, keep me motivated to continue the practice. More forgiveness results in more space in my being and in my life to be filled with divine light and love and magic.

And so, like the Greeks, I honor the new life that is burgeoning all around and within me by bowing inward and asking myself for the gift of this beautiful practice of forgiveness.

<u>Heart Healing Practices for Forgiveness</u>

Altar: Create an altar to forgiveness. Incorporate any objects that you associate with a person or situation you would like to forgive. Spend time with your altar, opening your heart to the possibility of forgiveness and perhaps doing one or more of the following forgiveness practices:

Forgiveness Practice for the Mind: Bring to mind a person or situation that you would like to forgive. Allow your thoughts to flow, without judging them. Witness the amount of thoughts that contain beliefs and agreements about the way things "should" have been. Notice any Judge-Victim patterns existing within these thoughts. Next, breathe deeply into your heart. Send energy from your heart to your mind, imagining your own love bathing your thoughts.

Forgiveness Practice for the Emotions: Sit in a quiet, contained place where you feel safe and comfortable. Focus your awareness of a person or situation that you would like to forgive. Allow your emotions to flow, simply witnessing them arise, exist, and fall away. Next, breathe deeply into your heart. Picture your own love radiating outward from your heart to your entire being.

Forgiveness Practice for the Energy Body: Focus on a person or situation that you would like to forgive. Observe your energetic reaction to this person or situation. Notice if there are places in your energy body that feel agitated, drained, or edgy or if there seem to be "holes" in your energy body in response to this person or situation. Direct energy from your heart to these locations, allowing your own love to be the substance that fuels your fire.

Forgiveness Practice for the Physical Body: Become aware of any places in your physical form where you may be storing grudges. Are there places in your body that respond to the mere thought of a person or situation you are having difficulty forgiving? If so, breathe deeply into your heart and direct the healing balm of your own love to those physical locations. With each breath, imagine the energy of your heart healing and renewing your physical form.

Celebrating Spring Renewal

In your body is the garden of flowers.
Take your seat on the thousand petals of the lotus, and
there gaze on the Infinite Beauty.
~ Kabir

The act of gathering together to celebrate Spring and all the new birth it brings has been an important activity of communities throughout the globe for millennia. The exact customs may differ between peoples and time periods, but the focus always remains the same: groups of people joining together in honor of the Earth's fertility. In communion, we plant flowers, paint and hide eggs, and enjoy feasts; we perform any rites and rituals that signify new birth. We give gratitude that the dark, cold season has passed and celebrate the cycle of death and rebirth that occurs with the turning of Winter into Spring.

The same is true when we work with our own personal Spring Renewals. We have been in periods of transition ~ between jobs, relationships, homes, phases of our life; these transitions echo that experienced on our beautiful planet each year. Whatever has been released, we honor its passing and celebrate the space that it leaves for new birth and new life.

Like the earth, many of us spend the darker times in our lives ~ whether they be actual Winter seasons or metaphoric "winters of the soul" ~ turning inward. Just as the earth is not "dead" during winter, we are not gone or even merely resting; instead, we are in a sort of pregnant phase ~ a time when things may be growing underneath the surface, even as we appear on the outside to be very still and calm. Although our bodies may be somewhat dormant, they are doing very hard work, very important work. No, it is not the work of Summer, which is active and obvious and full of fiery passion. It is the work of Winter, of nurturing things that are growing under the surface. The process of turning inward, of assessing whatever is transitioning in our lives, is vitally important to our personal growth, just as Winter hibernation is essential for plants and animals.

Winter is the season for cleaning and clearing to prepare for the beautiful new life forms that will be born in spring. As old plants and roots die and are composted, they become the very nutrients that will nourish the seeds germinating in the soil they share. Imagine a piece of land where nothing ever died. It would not take long before the roots of everything became entangled and began to suffocate themselves and one another.

We can see the same thing happening in our own lives. If we keep planting and planting, forever adding new intents and relationships and jobs and homes and never releasing the old ones, we suffocate all the life out of each of these things.

One absolutely essential component of birth is death – we must let go of things in order to welcome other things into our lives. And this letting go can be really challenging. Sometimes we tend to tightly cling onto things, both physical objects and more illusive but equally important habits and even beliefs, fearing that we will be lost without them; we grasp firmly onto these items, because we believe on some level that we *are* them.

When we align with life, we are given charge of our fields in all forms. We must plant and nourish the new life as well as clear out the old. The difficulty is that sometimes we cannot see that the plant we have loved for so long would actually benefit us so much more if it were compost. From our vantage point, it may look so healthy; but some greater source of wisdom can see that that beautiful plant no longer fits within this ecosystem.

And if our commitment has been to make room for new life, that plant has to go. The same is true of all the components ~ the jobs, relationships, homes, ways of being in the world ~ of our own ecosystems.

Heart healing practices are of great service as we heal and renew our relationship with our bodies, minds, and souls. Throughout this process, each of us has been preparing our fields for what we will plant this Spring.

This transition into a new Spring in our lives ~ whatever form that takes ~ calls for great celebration. After the challenges of "Winter times", we desire to honor that signs of life are returning. I invite you to actively celebrate all the transitions in your life by both honoring what is dying and helping birth that which is coming into form.

Every person, situation, and period of our lives has an important purpose, just as every living being on our planet has a purpose. We are wise to honor each of those people, situations, and periods as they pass, to celebrate the blessings and gifts they bestowed upon us, even as we release them to create space for blessings and gifts yet unknown. We can create memorials to these people, relationships, and situations as a way to offer gratitude for their presence in our lives. Even the most challenging times provide gifts; indeed, often the gifts born of the challenging "Winter" periods are often the most profound. And gratitude expressed for these gifts provides an enormous amount of heart healing.

Equally important is to honor that which is being born into our lives, to actively welcome these new births and to nurture their growth. Whether our Spring Renewals take the form of a new relationship with our body or a new physical home in which to rest our body, a season of retirement after a long career or a shifting relationship with someone close to us, they should be heralded with great joy and excitement.

Just as each Spring blossoms burst forth after long periods of growth in the cold, dark Earth, we all experience new birth throughout our entire lifetimes. When we focus our awareness on actively cultivating our fields, clearing them of old debris, and planting and nurturing the new life they will produce, we experience our own Spring Renewal.

It is my sincerest hope that we each journey through all the seasons of our lives with hearts wide open and receptive to all the beauty and love being showered upon us.

Heart Healing Practices for Celebration

Altar: Create an altar to your Heart Healing and Spring Renewal. Incorporate any objects that you associate with this healing and renewal. Spend time with your altar, connecting with your intent for healing and renewal.

Nature as Teacher: Dedicate some time to celebrating Spring Renewal in Nature. Delight in the evidence that renewal is always occurring in the natural world and receive and wisdom and teachings that may be important to you.

Sitting Practice: Breathe deeply into your heart. Take time to scan the different aspects of your being one by one: your mental body, energetic body, emotional body, and physical body. Witness the ways that you have created healing and renewal throughout your entire being. Allow your own love and gratitude to radiate outward from your heart to all parts of you.

Celebrate: Plan a celebration of your Spring Renewal. Design a ritual, hold a party, create a work of art ~ do anything you would like to celebrate Heart Healing your Body, Mind, and Soul.

Acknowledgments

This volume began as a series of articles I created to encourage myself through a period of great transition. Three Springs later, as I am emerging from one of the deepest Winter periods I have experienced, it is being birthed in an entirely new form. As with all new creations, indeed all transitions, it is only possible with the support of countless people. I am immensely grateful to the members of my tribe, both near and far, who inspire and guide me every single day.

To my beloved sweetheart, Raven Smith ~ You saw a book in a group of my writings, you saw a magical adventurous home in a poorly written internet advertisement, and you see love and light everywhere you look. It is an honor and a delight to share both my path and my life with you.

To my amazing children, Owen and Grace Zielinski ~ What a privilege it is to be your mother and to witness each of your amazing transformations.

To their wonderful father, John Zielinski ~ My depth of appreciation and admiration for who you are and what we share is limitless.

To Karen Wallace ~ Your beautiful talent enfolds this volume, just as your beautiful love enfolds the lives of so many of us.

To those who care for my physical heart, Heidi Connolly, Marvin Peyton, Hartzell Schaff, and hundreds of other doctors, nurses, and medical technicians ~ Thank you for helping to keep me alive.

To those who help care for my heart in all other ways, Gabriel Haaland, Adriana Magdalene, Laura Toups, Talya Ring, Tenaya Asan, Christine Steffien, Kevin Anthony Flores, Jai Cross, Micah Riot, Therese van Buskirk, Josianne Bischofberger, Marla Kaya, Juniper Park, Kim Christensen, Suzanne McBride, Arielle Webb, Jim Morris, Rhonda Reynolds, Laura Guzman, Mary Beth Fletcher, Lois Berdaus Hughs, Jim Gardner, Diane Osborne, Catherine Anderson, Lynda Griebenow, Tom McGarrity, Larry Winters, Jim Hickman, and so many more ~ Thank you for helping me live.

And to Michael, always to Michael.

Author Biography

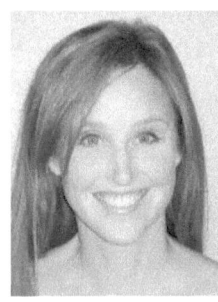

"I am a spiritual life coach, teammate, and cheerleader; a writer, reader, student, teacher. I am a seeker and journeyer, and my travels take me into all realms, most importantly that of infinite possibility."

Amy Zielinski has extensive experience as an archaeologist and art historian specializing in Ancient Mediterranean religious sites and objects, particularly those related to women's rituals. Her doctoral work, which focused on transition rites of young girls in Ancient Greece, instilled in her a desire to use ceremony and ritual to support contemporary people going through any of life's transitions. She is passionate about sharing her knowledge and enthusiasm with others through her ministry, teaching, and coaching. To find out more about the work Amy is doing please visit www.divineunion.us

Amy's Coaching

Spiritual life coaching is an amazing gift to give yourself. We all know the difficulty in changing the habitual behaviors that don't serve us, and in taking on successful actions that really support our desire to live a fuller, abundant, and peaceful life. A life coach offers incredible support and reflection that can keep us on track with our real goals in life.

Most importantly a good coach keeps us inspired. Doing great things with our life doesn't have to be a chore! It should be a joy to be living and manifesting our lives highest purpose. Having someone in your court that can keep you from grinding down and gritting your teeth, instead supporting you in staying charged up and excited with life is invaluable. We can all use a good cheerleader in our life, someone who supports us no matter what the obstacle and celebrates our successes and joys with us.

To get more information about coaching or to sign up for a session with Amy please email her at: amy.sacredspace@gmail.com

www.ingramcontent.com/pod-product-compliance
Lightning Source LLC
Chambersburg PA
CBHW032028290526
45786CB00011B/1052